Detox Diet
Eliminate Toxins, Rejuvenate Your Body, Look and Feel Great

Steven Ballinger

Legal Disclaimer

Important Insight

Detox diets have quickly gained a large following over the years, and as far as diets go, this one is here to stay. It is very popular because of its simplicity, its short duration, its benefits and the fact that it is natural and there are no chemicals or pills involved.

Detoxification is the body's natural way of eliminating toxins which cause harm to the body's tissues, which inevitably leads to a host of other issues such as infections, nutritional deficiency, inefficient metabolism, hormonal imbalance and other diseases.

The results of such physiological impairment lead to poor concentration, indigestion, muscle pain, skin problems, fatigue, bad breath, headaches, and sluggishness.

Furthermore, to aid the body's detox process, the diet includes eating or drinking mostly raw organic foods that help provide antioxidants, vitamins, nutrients and a lot of fiber.

If you pay much attention to healthy eating, then you know how popular detox diets have become. You may also have heard how hard they are to maintain and that this sort of diet requires a great deal of discipline. However, if you can stick to it, the benefits are tremendous.

All the information provided herein is aimed at keeping you healthy. You will find comprehensive detoxification that will blend well with you and your family's busy schedule.

1: What is Detox Diet?

Detoxification which is also referred in short form as detox is the body's ongoing process of eliminating toxins from different organ systems. Toxins are waste products that originate from normal cell activity such as homocysteine, lactic acid, ammonia and human made toxins.

When toxins are allowed to accumulate in body tissues, they may become potentially harmful to the body and this may result to onset of various degenerative diseases such as cancer, arthritis, heart diseases, obesity, high blood pressure, stroke, diabetes among others.

The liver, blood, skin, lungs, kidneys, intestines and lymphatic systems work synergistically to ensure that various toxins in the body systems are transformed chemically to less harmful state before being eliminated from the body.

Although body detox is primarily considered as a rehabilitation measure for drug and alcohol dependence, it can also be regarded as a program of herbs and special diets that remove dietary and environmental toxins from the body systems.

Detox diet plan can be a short term or long-term program. It is aimed at reducing the amount of chemicals ingested, emphasizes on healthy foods that are rich in vitamins, phytonutrients, antioxidants, minerals, complex carbohydrates, healthy fats and proteins. Such foods will help the body in detoxification.

Apart from emphasizing on consumption of healthy foods, a detox diet also insist on eating organic fruits and vegetables that will supply the body with essential nutrients.

Detox diet is basically formulated to eliminate toxins and oxidants absorbed by the body systems from consuming unhealthy foods that are high in preservatives, additives, artificial colors and cholesterol.

Due to the use of herbicides and pesticides among other chemicals in our gardens, our foods have become contaminated with chemicals that once in the system pose the risks of various diseases.

Formulating a detox diet plan that is rich in nutrients, the body will be able to adjust and eliminate various toxins. This will eventually lead to a healthy lifestyle.

Individuals who need to consider a detox diet are those who significantly consume high amount of foods that are rich in flavors, artificial colors, preservatives and additives and those who consume adequate amount of caffeine or alcohol.

Individuals who live in a polluted area, those who are recovering from viral or bacterial diseases and those who manifest irritability due to physical problems like stress, fatigue, skin irritation or skin lesions should definitely consider detox diet.

In addition to the above mentioned individuals, it is important to consider detox diet plan if you are experiencing black circles around the eyes, bloating around the stomach, abnormal muscle growth, bulging of the muscles in different parts of the body, recurring bowel disturbance or tired puffy eyes. This is important since a good dose of detox diet will help to ease such health concerns.

However, do not wait until you fall sick. According to research, many individuals in today's society are suffering from stomach ulcers, liver diseases, obesity, diabetes, irritable bowel syndrome among other general illness.

This is because we no longer consume organic foods that have reduced chemicals but instead we are consuming foods that are rich in saturated fats, high calories, added sugars, preservatives and high carbohydrates content.

For this reasons, we end up with much body complications which we are not able to comprehend. To avoid such problems, you need a detox diet that has well formulated meal plan so as to supply your body with nutrients that will facilitate detoxification.

After following a detox diet plan, an individual usually experience increased concentration, improved digestion, improved bowel movements, healthy skin and improved energy.

It is essential for any interested individual to follow the program strictly as outlined in this book. However, as a beginner you may notice certain side effects such as headaches which may occur due to caffeine withdrawal. Therefore, it is important before abiding to a detox diet program to first reduce the amount of caffeine and alcohol intake.

Other early symptoms include irritability, acne, tiredness, hunger and weight loss. Fortunately, such symptoms are short lived and will disappear within the first few days of following a detox diet plan.

2: Types of Detox Diet

Detox diets, also known as cleansing diets help in detoxification of the body in a healthy and natural way. There are two types of detoxification diets available today; short term and long term.

However, the basic concept of all these diets is that they should include natural foods which are high in vitamins, minerals and proteins. A healthy detoxification diet should have fiber.

Dietary fiber is essential for the smooth functioning of the digestive system that helps remove toxins from the body. Fibrous foods include nuts, oats, vegetables, fruits, wheat, brown rice and so forth. Here are the different types of detox diets available today;

Raw Food Diet

This diet consists of raw unprocessed food, fruits, dried fruits and leafy vegetables. These raw foods can be consumed through various methods like salads, juices or smoothies. Flavors can be added to make them tasty especially for the juices and smoothies.

During this diet, one should totally avoid any dairy products, cookies, pasta, meat, bread and deep fried fruits. Eating raw foods helps to prevent the loss of minerals, vitamins or any other essential elements that are lost through cleaning or cooking.

The good thing about eating uncooked food is the fact that it contains good potassium to sodium ratios which enhance cell functioning and pH balance. This is the overall objective of detox diets.

Master Cleanse Diet

This is certainly the most popular detox diet. It consists of maple syrup, lemonade and cayenne pepper. It enhances blood circulation in a very healthy way. The lemon juice helps to dissolve waste matter in the colon.
The maple syrup provides energy while the cayenne pepper gets rid of mucus in the body. This diet should be taken for ten days and one should not consume any solid foods, but just liquids.

Fresh Fruit Diet

This diet is very fresh and tasty. It consists of fresh fruits only and there is a wide variety of fruits to choose from. Any fruit is quite okay, but citrus fruits are highly recommended. There is also mono fruit detoxification product that involves the consumption of just one type of fruit.

The good thing about this diet is that it can be done over a long period of time because fruits supply the body with healthy water and allows the cells to clean. Fruits leave the human body's pH level more stable and make the sugar levels in the blood less erratic.

Green Smoothie Diet

This is also another popular form of a detox diet. It includes a miracle combination of vegetables and fruits. They are blended together in green smoothies to prepare nourishing healthy drinks. Blending vegetables also makes digestion easier without the loss of nutritional values.

Liver Cleansing Diet

The theory behind the invention of this detox diet is that the liver gets overloaded with waste products if it's not cleaned on a regular basis. For liver cleansing, mainly veggies, fruits, poultry and fish are consumed.

Drinking eight to twelve glasses of water daily is highly recommended. Healthy fats like avocado, salmon and virgin olive oil are included in this diet. The idea behind this diet is to make the liver function better and aid in weight loss. It is an eight-week program that ensures elimination of unhealthy foods from the diet.

Hallelujah Diet

For many people, eating raw foods three times a day can be difficult. This is where the Hallelujah diet comes in. It involves eating 85% raw food and 15% cooked food. The portion of cooked food should be consumed at the end of dinner.

One should also skip breakfast and consume beverages instead of vegetables and barley juices. To get the body adjust to life without breakfast, one can start by replacing eggs with fresh fruits, almond milk, multi-grain granola or toast with almond butter.

Although this detox diet does not reduce fat, it helps the body fluid. This information can be obtained from herbs and plants like asparagus, celery seed, dandelion, juniper berries, artichokes, watercress, parsley and melon.

Martha's Vineyard Detox

In this diet, only specialized vegetable and fruit liquids are ingested for a period of 21 days. There are also some solids taken. The combination of these fruit and vegetable drinks cleanses the body exceptionally well.

Fat Flush Diet

This is both a weight loss and detox diet. The idea behind it is to provide all the ingredients necessary to boost metabolism, promote fat loss and reduce water retention. It contains all the elements of a healthy and good weight loss program and runs in three phases.

Sugar Detox Diet

This diet was designed to help people kick out the sugar habit and have a more youthful appearance. It is a three-day detox plan that helps to get sugar out of the body system. In the three days, all forms of sugar are prohibited. The foods recommended are healthy fats and vegetables, whole grains, lean proteins, and legumes. In this period all strenuous activity should be avoided. Walking and yoga are the best exercises.

David Kirsch's 48 HR Supercharged Cleanse

This detox diet touts on the motto, "If you are chewing, then you are cheating". It's a two day cleanse that consists of subsisting several glasses of drink with ingredients like milk thistle, cranberry extract, acai berry and more. This detox promises to kick start the metabolism and cleanse the system.

Colon Detox Diet

Colon cleansing involves two paths; either through colon irrigation which pumps out water through the rectum by a colon therapist then flushes out the water and toxins, or through supplements like laxatives and teas which push out toxins from the colon.

Juju Detox Diet

This is a short blast program where dieters can choose from a one day to three day cleanse according to the level of juices ordered. These juices cannot be made at home, however, the ingredients include, carrots, ginger, pineapple, beets, honey, lemon and ginger.

All these are types of detox diets that one can choose from. The effectiveness of a detox type depends on one's body, current health and the motivation to stick to the selected plan. They require a user to design their lives around a strict meal plan with set timings. For people with other obligations that require more flexibility, the right diet type might be difficult to find.

3: Why You Need a Detox Diet Now

Get toxins out of your body

What with water treatment plants, food processing taking place under the nose of the Food and Drug Administration, you might think that food and drinks are healthier than they have ever been before.

However, just walking outside exposes you to environmental pollutants, and the cleansers, dyes, fabrics and other substances we touch everyday have chemicals that are harmful.

Even taking your dog for a walk to the park exposes you to all the pesticides that your city uses to keep the bugs at bay. These chemicals lodge in cells and tissues all over your body, even in your brain, and they stay there for years. Detox diet helps these substances find their way out of your body faster.

Keep chronic diseases away

The toxins in the environment are the root causes for many of the cancers and neurological conditions out there. Stroke and heart disease are two other by products of exposure to these substances. It is true that each of us has a detox system inside us - the liver and the rest of the endocrine system.

However, the load of toxins coming in each day overloads that system. Detoxing helps your body do what it is built to do naturally - get those toxins out of your system.

Drop those unwanted pounds

Many toxins hinder the body's natural propensity to burn fat. If you add those to the increasingly sedentary lifestyle that most people already lead, you're talking about a weight gain epidemic that is even more dangerous. When your weight gets out of control, high blood pressure, type 2 diabetes and heart disease all become ominous possibilities.

When you detox, you get rid of the toxins that are lurking in your fat cells, and you boost your metabolism, making it easier to keep that weight down.

Increase your levels of energy

If you have ever seen someone consume poison in a movie, you see how quickly it brings all of their bodily functions to a halt. The toxins that you take in from the environment are not large enough in volume to have that quick of an effect, but over time, the buildup of toxins in your system robs you of your energy.

When you detox, those substances are no longer in your system slowing you down. As a result, you feel higher levels of energy and have an improved quality of life.

Slow down the aging process

Have you ever wondered why pictures of coal miners from the 1800s showed men who looked 50 or 60 years old, even though they were lucky if they made it to the age of 40?

The buildup of coal dust in the lungs, along with time spent working in conditions not allowing them to stand up straight, accelerated their aging process significantly. By the time they were 40, these men had lungs that were simply full of black, tarry dust that made even simple breathing a real trial.

Most of us don't work in coal mines today, but we walk around in an environment that is full of pesticides, toxic emissions from industry and other pollutants. Breathing those substances in contributes to our aging process by inhibiting our ability to absorb nutrients as well. A detox reverses that process, slowing the aging clock down once again.

Boost the function of your immune system

If your immune system is too busy fighting off toxins, it won't be able to do much when viruses like the flu and the common cold sets in. If you're always fighting off a cold or you have the flu every winter, your quality of life begins to suffer. Over time, becoming sick regularly becomes a vicious cycle. When you detox regularly, your immune system works more efficiently, keeping infections from taking hold.

Give yourself happier skin

The skin is your first line of defense when you walk out the door every morning, and toxins in the environment often hit the skin first - even before they hit our lungs. Pores end up getting clogged, leading to outbreaks of acne. Poor absorption of nutrients leads to nails and hair that are brittle and weak.

Detoxing regularly makes nails and hair stronger, and your skin can deal with the oils that lead to acne more effectively. As a result, you will walk around with a healthy aura about yourself.

Give your body its balance back

The human nervous, digestive and hormonal systems work with one another to bring about the best overall health. Your body wants to be healthy, and its natural processes are designed to keep everything running smoothly.

When you take in too many foods that are not healthy and immerse your body in toxins, these systems simply can't work as well. The end result is that we feel sick (or at least have a lack of energy). Detoxing brings back that balance.

When the systems in the human body are aligned properly, you also notice a shift in your emotional and mental condition. It is easier to make difficult decisions and endure tough situations. Analyzing confusing situations becomes easier, and you feel like a cloud has lifted from your entire day.

Putting a detox diet to work for you is an excellent way to improve your body's physical health while also giving your entire life a fresh reboot. Beginning a detox diet is not easy at first, but the benefits are more than worthwhile. Talk to your physician if you have concerns about your own situation, but by and large, detox diets are safe and effective.

4: Ways to Eliminate Toxins in Your Body

Toxins are substances or chemicals which cause harm to the cells and organs in the body as well as their everyday functions. They are divided into two groups; those that are created internally, especially by undigested and over-processed foods that create a toxic build up and those from an outside source that are ingested or inhaled.

The body produces toxic trash metabolites which must be cleared. They could cause serious health problems if one has digestive problems, fatigue, sinus problems, or recovering from an accident or an injury if they are not cleared properly.

To ensure that the body is working optimally, it is essential to have the toxins eliminated from the body on a regular basis. There are four main removal systems that work in harmony with each other to accomplish this. They include;

1. The disposal of all cellular waste products but especially lactic acid.

2. The removal of large waste products through the lymph. The smaller waste products go the veins and are sent or exhaled to the liver.

3. The processing of the toxins by the liver. Most of these go into the bile duct and then into the digestive tract for final removal. The water soluble ones go to the kidneys to be excreted as urine.

4. The last clearance of the waste products by the digestive tract.

Here are a few tips that you could follow to eliminate toxins in your body;

Reduce Your Toxin Intake

This is without a doubt the first step to toxin elimination. It is quite self defeating to completely eliminate toxins when you are still taking in a significant amount of them. Switch to organic beverages and foods and drink distilled or filtered water. Avoid all products that could contain toxins like inorganic perfumes and cosmetics and avoid exposure to airborne chemicals and cigarette smoke.

Green Grapes

Have plenty of green grapes each day. They contain detoxifying qualities and draw out any toxins from all organs in the body and dump them into the intestines for elimination. They are also rich in fiber so they will ensure that digestion is done properly. Since they contain some juice, they are highly recommended for people who are not able to take so many glasses of water each day.

Sweat It Out

The skin is the biggest organ in the body and one of the main organs responsible for elimination. Baths, steam rooms and saunas are good detoxification aids since they increase perspiration. They can eliminate up to 20% of debris and toxins from the body through the skin.

Exercise

Have a routine exercise for at least thirty minutes each day. Without exercise, the lymphatic system becomes stagnant and causes waste to accumulate in the body. The lymphatic system ensures that the immune system is working at its peak. Exercise also increases sweating and we all know that sweating effectively gets rid of toxins from the body.

Stretches

Stretches will kick up your detox efforts. Stretching allows oxygenated blood to all part of the body while carrying out any toxins with it. Exercises like tai chi and yoga are great exercises that incorporate stretching.

Evacuate

Evacuate to remove debris and dirt from all the organs in the body. If you do not eliminate properly, your efforts are in vain. Having two to three bowel movements everyday is vital in the elimination of waste. If you are not doing this, you could consider a mild herbal supplement like triphala, magnesium to help you.

Full Body Rub

Treat yourself to rubs with organic sea salt occasionally. Salts contain detoxifying qualities which increase perspiration. They also exfoliate the skin to get rid of skin cells and dirt that could be blocking skin pores. Skin pores play a vital role in the detoxification process.

Water

Water is very important in toxin removal. Drink eight to twelve glasses of water everyday to speed up kidney activities and increase the removal of toxins. You could incorporate vinegar, cayenne pepper and lemon to your water. These components increase your metabolism and energy and also clear toxins and mucus from all vital organs. Water also prevents constipation that could be caused by the increased fiber intake.

Get rid of processed and gluten foods

Processed foods do not contain any nutrients. So when you consume them, you are only eating artificial stuff. They include gluten, wheat protein, which causes a sluggish metabolism and hence accumulation of toxins inside the body.

Avoid Sugar

Sugar is very hard to digest and messes the blood sugar levels. Since it is not readily digestible, it accumulates in the body as toxins. It might be very hard to kick the sugar habit, however, try to steer away from artificial sweeteners and refined sugars.

Detox Tea

Dandelion, neem and goldenseal are some of the best detox herbal teas. You can also make some tea with turmeric powder. If you prefer pill supplements, you could try the milk thistle.

Vitamin D and Fresh Air

Vitamin D is essential to the overall health. Go outside and maximize time under the sun. Breathe in as much fresh air as possible too while at it.

Deep Breaths

We underestimate the cleansing power of deep breaths and therefore don't forget to breathe deeply and consciously. When you wake up in the morning, take around eight to ten minutes to breathe deeply. This is very cleansing and invigorating.

Sleep

Ensure to get more sleep everyday. Although it might not be responsible for cleansing the body itself, it is incredibly important for maintaining the normal body functions and the overall well being.

5: Detox Diet Plan: The Do's and Don'ts

The detox diet has become popular as more people begin to understand just how much toxins their bodies accumulate through day to day activities. Toxins are present in air, water and food.

Common ways in which people ingest toxins are through antibiotics, hormones present in food, pesticides, detergents, food additives, drugs, cigarette smoke and many more. Combine this with a daily diet lacking in nutrients, and you will find that the body's natural ability to get rid of these toxins is impaired.

Armed with this new information on the impact toxins and poor diet can have on your body, you may have already made the decision to make use of a detox diet consistently. In fact, you probably already have a few recipes on hand that you cannot wait to try out.

However, before you do, it is important for you to read the top do's and don'ts of a detox diet. The tips below are like a basic guideline of what you should and shouldn't do during a detox diet plan.

Do's

1. ***Do talk to your doctor or physician*** – despite the fact that a detox diet is natural and has numerous health benefits for the body, it is always important that you first consult with your physician about undertaking a new diet.

2. ***Do a lot of exercises*** – exercises help further boost the natural process of detoxification. Aside from aiding you in losing some pounds, exercise helps detoxification by stimulating blood flow, respiration and lymphatic flow.

   Additionally, exercising also helps in strengthening and boosting the functions of the kidney, liver, lungs and digestive tract that are all responsible for getting rid of toxins in the body.

3. **Do drink a lot of water** - the whole process of eliminating toxins from the body requires a lot of water, so it is encouraged that you drink at least half of your weight in ounces, of water daily.

4. ***Do a lot of research*** – before you embark on any detox diet plan, you need to research on a variety of things such as the kind of detox diet you want to start, what food to eat or what food to avoid, the health benefits of the ingredients of the detox diet, and whether or not that particular detox diet will meet your goals.

Don'ts

1. ***Don't overdo it*** – too much of a good thing can become bad. If you are just starting out on your first detox diet, it is advised that you do it for a maximum of 2 days. This is because your body may not be able to handle a 10 day detox diet plan, especially if it is the first time. Start out small, and once you get the hang of it, increase the number of days gradually.

2. ***Don't overindulge*** – It is quite obvious that you should be able to maintain a healthy diet and lifestyle during the detox diet, but it is important that you carry out these changes and practices even before or after the detox

diet. You would simply be negating the effects of the detox diet by indulging in foods or a lifestyle that is full of toxins.

3. ***Don't stress*** – during your detox diet, it is important for you to try to maintain a relaxed state of mind. High levels of stress will only cause your body to use up a lot of vitamin B and C which are important to the body's detoxification process. It will inevitably lead to a poor detoxification process, and possibly a health risk situation. If possible, incorporate different stress-releasing techniques in your daily routine.

4. ***Don't stay up late*** – ancient detoxification practices state that the body's detoxification process is strongest between the hours of 9pm and midnight. If possible, during your detox diet, aim to sleep during this period of time and avoid any activities that may require you to stay up late.

The above mentioned tips are simply guidelines meant for you to follow during your detox diet plan. They can be tweaked to suit your own preferences. This means that there are numerous detox diets for you to choose from.

As you go through the different diet plans, always ensure that whatever ingredients are included are ones that you can easily find at your local organic food store, and that they are fresh and in season. This means you can make use of fruits and vegetables that are readily available.

Aside from the abundance, this will also help you save money in the long run that you would have otherwise spent on searching for and buying exotic fruits and vegetables shipped from across the world, simply because the detox diet plan states that they should be included.

It is also important for you to always remember that what may work for someone else, may not work for you. Listen to your body, and if it likes a certain detox diet plan, stick to it, and avoid jumping on a bandwagon of a diet just because everyone else is.

6: Colon, liver and kidney cleansing diet

Colon, also known as large intestine, is one of the major organs in the body responsible for waste removal. Experts estimate that there are over 100 trillion friendly bacteria residing in the colon.

Unhealthy eating habits, lack of exercise and stress lead to an unhealthy colon. A diet full of adequate nutrients, fiber and water will result in a clean and healthy colon.

For effective colon cleanse, your diet should be rich in fiber as fiber helps in cleaning the debris formed by the remnants of food left behind in the colon during the waste removal.

Green foods are rich in chlorophyll which helps in healing the digestive tract. You also need to include some fermented foods such as yogurt as it replenishes the friendly bacteria in your colon. Also, drink a lot of pure water to keep your body clean and free of toxins.

Since colon works as a fuelling station as well as a waste management center, during the cleaning process a mixture of bile acids, bacteria and fungi and other toxins is left behind. All of these put together create debris in the colon. A plant based diet is necessary for effective colon cleansing. We take a look at some of the foods which should be included in your diet for effective colon cleansing.

Foods Rich in Fiber

A high-fiber diet is necessary for a healthy colon. Fiber comes in both soluble and insoluble varieties. Soluble fiber is responsible for increasing the quantity of beneficial bacteria in the body.

The beneficial bacteria help in removing other harmful bacteria from the body such as salmonella and E. coli. Soluble fiber also helps in bringing down the cholesterol levels in the body by binding with it and helping it pass through the body.

Insoluble fiber helps in sweeping the debris in the colon similar to a broom. It also helps in exercising the large intestine by helping it produce wavelike muscular contractions.

These muscular contractions help in decreasing the bowel transmit time as well as toning the muscle. Another benefit of fiber is that it retains water in the colon which helps in softening the stool.

Rich sources of soluble fiber are rice, citrus, strawberry, barley, peas, beans and apples. Oats and flax seeds are also rich in soluble fiber. Insoluble fiber can be found in good quantities in cabbage, carrots, deeds, Brussels sprouts, turnips, cauliflower, wheat, rye, brown rice and apple with skin.

It is recommended to consume between 20 to 35 grams of fiber each day. You can consume five or more servings of fruits and vegetables to fulfill the daily requirement. Six or more servings of whole grains will also provide you with recommended fiber.

One serving of fruit or vegetable means a half cup of fruit or vegetables or one full cup of raw and leafy greens. As far as grains are concerned, one slice of bread or half cup of cooked pasta or cereal makes up one serving.

Chlorophyll Rich Green Foods

Chlorophyll helps in cleansing colon by healing the damaged tissue in the digestive tract. It also helps by retaining more oxygen in the body which in turn helps in flushing out more toxins.

Foods rich in chlorophyll are wheat grass, barley grass, spirulina, alfalfa and blue green algae.

Drink a Lot of Water

You must have read that water is a universal solvent. It means that it is the most powerful solvent known to humankind and it dissolves almost everything. Lack of water can result in constipation and increase the toxin levels in the body.

It is important to realize that caffeinated beverages or caffeinated drinks do not count as water as they are high in salt and sugar which leads to dehydration. A good rule of thumb is to drink anywhere from 8 to 10 glasses of water a day.

Fermented Foods

Fermented foods are a good source of friendly bacteria. These friendly bacteria help the body by stimulating the immune system, synthesizing vitamins from food, degrading the toxins, preventing disease causing bacteria and by producing fatty acids which are an important source of energy for the cells which line the colon.

For fermented foods, you should include yogurt, miso, sauerkraut and kefir in your diet. When consuming supermarket yogurt, make sure that you are not eating yogurt high in sugar as it will negate all the positives of yogurt.

Liver Cleansing Diet

There are many different liver cleansing diets available in the market. Some of the more radical liver cleansing diets recommend use of lemon juice, Epsom salts, olive oil, Cayenne Pepper and other such things. It is not recommended to use these ingredients as it may be harmful to your liver. However, you can certainly make other changes to your diet which will result in cleansing your liver naturally.

Your liver cleansing diet should include nuts, legumes, vegetables, seeds and high-fiber fruits in addition to pure water. Some of the foods which help in liver cleansing are carrots, onions, spinach, tomatoes, apples, beets, broccoli, walnuts, oat bran, spices such as turmeric and cinnamon, brown rice and Brussels sprouts.
You should avoid food rich in refined sugar and saturated fats. Also avoid alcohol.

Kidney Cleansing Diet

For cleansing your kidney properly, you need to include foods which are low in protein. Since high protein intake leads to build up of urea in the body, it puts stress on kidney for cleansing.

Meat, dairy products and seafood have high protein content and these should be avoided. Breads, grains, starches, fruits and vegetables have low protein content and these should be included in your diet. However, it is important to consume adequate quantity of protein to have a balanced diet.

In addition to a low protein diet, you should also avoid foods rich in phosphorus. Since weakened kidneys are not able to remove phosphorus effectively from the blood, a phosphorus rich diet will raise the level of phosphorus in blood which can lead to calcium loss.

For optimum kidney cleansing, your diet should include potatoes, pumpkin, watermelon, celery, cucumber, legumes, seeds, parsley, and algae products such as spirulina, blue green algae and chlorella.

If your kidney is not functioning properly, it is also possible that your body may become deficient in some particular vitamins and minerals. Therefore, after checking with your healthcare provider, you may consume supplements of vitamins C, B complex, vitamin D3 and calcium.

A healthy colon, liver and kidney are vital to your overall health. Effective colon, Liver and Kidney cleansing is possible by making some diet changes. Therefore, create a diet based on the ingredients given above and keep your body healthy and free of toxins.

7: Fruit and Vegetable Detox Recipes

Even the most health fanatics are aware of the instances when they have strayed away from their healthy regimes more often than they would like to stick to them. Holidays, weekends and vacations are perfect example, where steel-cut oatmeal and almonds are replaced by penne and bacons in breakfast, and fresh fruits have no place in the meal plans.

Once you are done with your vacationing, you might start feeling fatigue, leading to headaches and feeling of laziness throughout the day. What is that? Well, it is a sign that you have stuffed your body with too much toxins and now you need to find a way to get rid of them in a natural way.

Detox Your Way To Healthy Living

A fresh fruit and vegetable detox diet can be a great way to boost your metabolism and immune system, as well as keep your digestive system healthy.

Juicing or juice recipes allow you to intake huge amount of fresh foods in the form of hard pressed juices. If you want to get rid of the body's toxins and lose a few pounds, a juice detox can be a great option.

Detox diet recipes are a great way to lose weight quickly, while removing toxins from your body. Most detox diets focus on a lot of fresh fruits, vegetables, water and juices.

Since fruit and vegetable detox recipes are very low in calories, you should be able to get multiple benefits from them.

The Clean Diet

The clean diet detox plan is based on having just 3 meals a day, which include two liquid and one solid meal. Indulging in nutrient rich organic fruits and vegetables is the focal point of this diet. The liquid meals consists of blends of fresh fruits and vegetables.

On the other hand, the solid meal can include salads and lean protein of choice. Foods allowed in this kind of plan include carrots, mango, cucumbers, pineapple, apples, melons, leafy green vegetables and blueberries.

Fruit Flush Diet

This is a 3 day detox diet that will help you lose weight up to ten pounds during the process. In the first day of the detox, you must drink a glass of juice every 2 hours. In the dinner, eat 3-6 cups of freshly chopped vegetables, a lean protein serving and 1-2 tablespoon flax seed oil.

In the next two days, you should include one serving of fresh fruits every 2 hours and one serving of vegetables in the dinner.

Detox Juice Recipes

Detox juice recipes play essential role in boosting your body's cleansing abilities. You can use any of your favorite fruit or vegetable to make the detox juice recipes.

However, if you have some specific goals in mind, you might want to try improving your knowledge about different benefits of fruits and vegetables. There are some specific foods that works well for cleansing. These are:

- Cucumbers and celery - Natural diuretics
- Beets - Work greatly for liver cleansing
- Lemons, ginger and apples - These aid in cleansing the entire body
- Cranberries - These are good for cleansing the bladder.

- Green vegetables - These nourish and clean our cells simultaneously.

Fruits and Vegetables Detox Recipes

Directions:

Cut all the ingredients in small chunks and blend together in a blender.
Add ½ - 1 cup of water or almond milk (unsweetened).

Carrot Cucumber Detox

- Carrots - 3-4
- Cucumber - 1
- Beet - 1/2
- Lemon - 1/2
- Gingerroot -1

Cucumber Beet Detox

- Cucumber - 1
- Carrots - 3
- Beet - 1
- Celery - 2 stalks
- Parsley - 1 handful
- Lemon - ½

Tomato Kick Detox

- Tomatoes - 2
- Green lettuce leaves - 2
- Radishes - 2
- Parsley sprigs - 4
- Lemon - ½

Vegetable Mix Detox

- Carrots - 3-4
- Celery stalks - 2
- Beet - 1/2
- Broccoli florets - 2
- Lemon - 1/2

Cucumber Apple Detox

- Fennel - 2 stalks of
- Cucumber - 1/2
- Green apple - 1/2
- Mint - 1 handful
- Gingerroot - 1 inch

Cabbage Salad Detox

- Green cabbage - 1 (quarter head)
- Carrots - 3

- Celery stalks - 4

Perfect Skin Juice Detox

- Cucumber - 1
- Parsnip - 1
- Carrots - 2-3
- Lemon - 1/2
- Green pepper - ¼

Total Body Detox Juice

- Tomato - 1
- Asparagus - 1
- Cucumber - 1
- Lemon - 1/2

Liver Cleanse Detox

- Dandelion - 1 handful
- Carrots - 3-4
- Cucumber - 1/2
- Lemon peeled - 1/2

Detox Vegetable Meal Recipes
Roasted Vegetable Recipe

Ingredients:

- Diced potato - 1
- Chopped bell pepper - 1
- Chopped raw mushrooms - 1
- Onion - 1
- Tomatoes - 1
- Pineapple chunks - 1
- Olive oil - 3 tbsp
- Chopped garlic - 2 tsp
- Dill weed - 2 tsp
- Celery salt - 1 tsp

Directions

- Chop all the vegetables into small sized chunks and place them in a large bowl.

- Place vegetables in a roasting pan and bake at 400 degrees.

- Stir for 10 minutes or until tender.

Vegan Mushroom Stuffed Mushrooms

Ingredients

- Portabella Mushroom caps - 2
- Mushrooms - 1 container (sliced)

- Onion - 1 small diced
- Tomatoes - 4 roma (diced)
- Tofu - 1/2 block lite (crumbled)
- Tomato sauce - 1/2 cup

Directions

- Saute all the vegetables until they are tender.

- Add tomato and tofu sauce

- You may also add some spices such as garlic powder, oregano, basil etc.

- Saute mushroom caps until properly cooked.

- Combine them and serve

Lemon Cilantro Eggplant Dip

- Eggplant - 2 pound each
- Cloves garlic - 3-4
- Tahini - 3 tablespoons
- Fresh lemon juice - 3 tablespoons
- Salt- to taste
- Cilantro or mint leaves - ¼ cups
- Toasted or grilled pita wedges

- Carrot and cucumber sticks

Directions

- Preheat oven at 450 degrees F.
- Line a 15" by 10" jelly roll pan with the nonstick foil
- Place eggplant halves with skin sides up..
- Wrap garlic in the foil and place into the pan with eggplants.
- Roast vegetables for about 45 to 50 minutes.
- Unwrap the garlic cloves.
- Cool garlic and eggplants until easy to handle.

When cool, scoop out the eggplant into the food processor. Squeeze out all the garlic pulp and add lemon juice, tahini, and salt. Cover and refrigerate for 2 hours. Serve dip with vegetables and pita.

8: Smoothie Detox Recipes

5 Reasons Why You Should Drink Green Smoothie

1. Boost your immune system - Daily intake of green vegetables supports optimal health and gives you more energy. Components found in green vegetables are the source that provides a healthy immune system.

2. Decreases the risk of cancer - Eating plenty of fruits and vegetables lowers the risk of stomach, esophagus, lung, pancreas, and colon cancer.

3. Lowers the risk of depression - consumption of fruits and vegetables on a daily basis significantly lowers the symptoms of depression.

4. Prevents diabetes - Daily intake of fruits and vegetables reduce the risk of diabetes. It also helps diabetes patients achieve well balanced diet.

5. Prevents heart disease - Eating plenty of fruits rich in vitamin C and leafy vegetables has a protective effect on the heart

Smoothie Recipes

Directions

1. Chop all ingredients into small chunks
2. Mix it in a blender
3. Drink

Beginner Green Smoothie

- 2 cup spinach
- 2 cup water
- 1 cup mango
- 1 cup pineapple
- 2 bananas

Simple Green Smoothie

- 2 cup water
- 3 banana
- 2 stalk celery
- 1 cup blueberry (fresh or frozen)
- 3 cup mixed green vegetable

Peach Coconut Smoothie

- 2 cup spinach
- 1 cup coconut water
- 2 cup peach
- 1 cup white seedless grapes

Green Tea Avocado Smoothie

- 16 oz. green tea
- ½ avocado
- ¼ teaspoon fresh ginger powder
- 1 banana
- 2 teaspoon honey
- 2 ice cubes

Cilantro Mango Smoothie

- 1½ spinach
- ½ cup Cilantro
- 2 cup water
- 1½ cup mango
- 1 cup pineapple
- ½ avocado

Green Smoothie (For healthy skin & Nail)

- ½ fresh lemon

- 1 apple
- 1 pear
- 1 stalk celery
- 1½ cup water
- 1 head romaine lettuce
- 1 cup spinach
- 1 banana

Chia Chia Smoothie

- 1 tablespoon chia seeds
- 1 cup almond milk (unsweetened)
- Soak it in milk for 15 minutes
- ¼ teaspoon nutmeg
- ¼ teaspoon cardamom
- ½ teaspoon cinnamon
- 1 pear
- 5 strawberries
- ½ orange
- 1 scoop protein powder
- 1½ cup baby kale or mixed green

Summer Smoothie

- 1/4 watermelon
- 2 cup strawberries

- 1 tablespoon lemon juice
- 1 lettuce
- Add water or almond milk

Energy booster smoothie

- 1 apple
- 1 banana
- 7 prunes
- 1cup spinach
- Add water or almond milk

Pomegranate Acai smoothie

- 2 cup frozen blueberries
- 2 ripe frozen banana
- 1/4 cup pomegranate juice
- 2 tablespoon acai berry juice
- Add water as needed

9: Top 10 Detox Super Foods

While detox is ongoing and natural, there are certain foods than bolster and even expedite the process, by providing nutrients, essential fatty acids, minerals and fiber as well as antioxidants. Basically, these foods help neutralize and eliminate environmental and dietary toxins from the body much faster.

Below is a comprehensive look at the top 10 detox super foods you must include in your diet if you want to keep your body healthy and free of toxins;

1. Cabbage

Regarded as one of the most affordable foods for detox, cabbage is laced with glucosinolates and compounds containing sulfur which the body converts into indoles and isothiocyanates. Isothiocyanates are known to eliminate carcinogens from the body thereby preventing cancer.

In addition, cabbage contains high volumes of vitamin C and fiber which cleanse the liver and regulate bowel movements respectively thus propelling harmful toxins out of the body.

Whenever possible, eat cabbage in its raw form as its active compounds are destroyed by heat. You can have it in salad, juice or as a smoothie.

2. Ginger

It's almost impossible to talk about detox foods without mentioning ginger. Ginger is a natural anti-inflammatory food that helps reduce nausea, enhance digestion and prop up detoxification by accelerating food movement through the intestines largely due to the presence of compounds known as shagoals and gingerols.
The best way to derive maximum detoxifying benefits of ginger is to use it as a salad dressing or making ginger juice and have it with vegetables.

3. Blueberries

Blueberries are full of vitamin C and fiber. At the same time they are low in calories and are rated as one of the super foods that have the highest antioxidant capacity.

The blue pigment of blueberries contains an antioxidant called anthocynanins which helps safeguard cells against free radical damage, boost production of glutathione and lower the chances of suffering from glaucoma, cataracts, diabetes, allergies and certain forms of cancer.

While it's easy to eat blueberries due to their taste, you can add a handful to your smoothie or cereal. You can use them to mask your vegetables or simply eat them as pudding after dinner.

4. Lemons

Lemons are without doubt one of the most potent foods for detox. They are chock-full of vitamin C and are thought to aid in restoration of alkaline-balance of the body thus making it possible for your body to get rid of environmental and dietary toxins. Lemons are natural energizers too and can help fight the symptoms of an upsurge of toxins in the body.

To fully enjoy its detoxifying benefits, squeeze half a lemon into a glass of warm water and drink the mixture religiously each morning before eating anything.

5. Apples

The good old adage that says an apple a day keeps the doctor away makes every sense, considering that apples contain high levels of insoluble and soluble pectin fiber which marinates harmful toxins and waste.

In addition apples are laced with glucaric sugar acid, which aids the body in removal of estrogen-like compounds and heavy metals.

You can either slice the apples to make a snack, use them as a dessert or simply eat the fruit for detox. You may consider adding sliced apples to a salad as well.

6. Beets

Beets have potassium, fiber and folate as well as antioxidants. The betaine contained in beets is known to lower levels of inflammation, protect the liver from damage in addition to helping it process fats.

The reddish-purple beets pigment is packed with betacyanin, an anti-inflammatory antioxidant which also supports detoxification. Beets are also low in calories; a half cup beet juice contains forty calories.

Add grated or sliced raw beets to a salad or a sandwich to get the most out of this super food. Beets juice can be added to smoothies or mixed with apples or ginger juice too.

7. Garlic

A detox choice for many people, garlic is amalgamated with sulfur which not only helps fight harmful bacteria in the intestines but bolsters the body's capacity to detox by speeding up the production of glutathione required for removal of certain toxins from the body.

A sulfur compound referred to as allicin, converted by the body to allyl sufides is thought to offer protection against certain cancers, diabetes, arthritis and heart disease.

You have to chop or crush garlic to relinquish the the power of its sulfur compounds. Add it to a salad dressing, lemon juice, olive oil or eat 2-4 cloves of garlic a day for detox.

8. Green Tea

Green tea might not be a food per se but will fit into any detox program thanks to its high antioxidant content. It contains powerful antioxidant compounds known as epigallocatechin-3-gallate (EGCG) that can help the body eliminate free radicals and oxidation of LDL cholesterol. EGCG also improves the liver's functionality which is important as far as detoxification is concerned.

You may consider drinking 2-3 cups of ginger tea either as iced tea or a hot beverage. Avoid drinking coffee, alcohol or soda when you're using green tea for detox.

9. Cauliflowers

Despite its look, cauliflower is high in phytochemicals known as glucosinolates. The body breaks down these phytochemicals in the intestines to indole-3 carbinol and isothiocynates, two important compounds responsible for regulating the body's detoxification enzymes in addition to offering protection against cancer.

To get the most out of cauliflower for your detox plan, chop the vegetable in a food processor then steam or use it as a substitute for mashed potatoes.

10. Avocados

The fat contained in avocados is monounsaturated, meaning it won't obstruct the balance of omega3 to 6 fatty acids in the diet. Fat is an important part of a detox diet, bearing in mind it enhances bile production from the gallbladder.

This in effect facilitates elimination of toxins from the body and promotes absorption of fat-soluble vitamins such as vitamins A, D, E and K. Besides containing desirable fat, avocados are rich in folate and potassium as well. One cup of avocado juice has 18 grams of dietary fiber.

To enjoy its benefits, you can add avocado in smoothies and salads or drink its juice.

We can hardly escape the exposure to toxins, not with the high levels of air, water and soil pollution. Therefore it's only reasonable if we assisted the liver and the gallbladder get rid of harmful toxin despite detoxification being a natural process. These 10 detox super foods will help do exactly that and would make a great addition to any detox plan or diet.

10: Using Herbs and Supplements for Detox

According to Thomas Carlyle, "He, who has health, has hope; and he, who has hope, has everything." A healthy lifestyle starts with a healthy body and a healthy body needs regular cleansing of harmful toxins. Our body has a natural capability of getting rid of these harmful chemicals; however, exposure to a large number of chemicals in our day-to-day activities has slowed down this cleansing process.

5 Signs that your body needs detoxification

The chemistry of our environment has changed drastically in the past few decades including chemical contamination of ground water. Food industry has witnessed an increase in chemical usage for preservation and added flavors. These chemicals tax our immune system and the adverse effects of these chemicals are quite visible on our body. Some common signs of high toxin level in your body include:

- Low energy levels
- Constipation, indigestion, stomach pain
- Seasonal allergies
- Weak immune system

- Difficulty in losing weight

What are the best methods for detoxification?

Detoxification is a circular process, which repeats itself every few days or even hours depending upon the type of excretion. Some of the best methods of detoxification are:

- Fasting; offers rest to the organs.
- Healthy nutrients in the diet to promote detoxification
- Detoxification through skin, kidneys and intestines
- Better blood circulation (exercises)
- Using herbs and supplements for detoxification

We are going to discuss the most effective and common method of detoxification i.e. Using herbs and supplements for detox. Most of the detox programs prefer the use of herbs for toxin removal and it is extremely popular among participants.

How herbs and supplements can help in detoxification?

Using herbs and supplements for detox is an age-old process and one can find its traces in different day-to-day rituals. Herbs have several unknown qualities including their capability to heal and detox our body from toxins. However, it is important to understand the different types of herbs you need for effective detoxification.

5 Herbs for promoting detoxification in the body

1. **Psyllium Husk**: Psyllium husk is known for its effectiveness in restoring your digestive system health including intestines and it keeps harmful bacteria at bay. It is extremely helpful for individuals suffering from constipation, indigestion, irritable bowel syndrome and diarrhea. One should take it with plenty of water and upon entering the body; it transforms into gelatin-like mass and scrubs off toxins from your intestines. It offers effective colon cleansing to your digestive system.

2. **Probiotics**: Probiotics are effective against toxins present in your gut and because of the regular use of GMOs (Genetically Modified

Organisms); your body loses its natural bacterial balance. Probiotics replenish healthy bacteria in your body and have an overall cleansing effect. Some rich sources of Probiotics include yogurt, fermented veggies, kombucha tea, miso soup, kefir and similar products.

3. ***Sacred Bark*** (Cascara Sagrada): Cascara Sagrada or Sacred Bark is one of the most effective colon-cleansing herbs and it is being used for bowl cleansing for last several centuries. It is responsible for provoking contraction in your intestinal walls and improves the strength of the muscles of your intestinal lining. In addition to these benefits, sacred bark has a laxative effect that helps in colon cleansing.

4. ***Burdock Root***: Burdock root is known for its blood-cleansing properties and it can remove dangerous chemicals including herbicide chemicals, pesticides, bacteria, parasites, blood toxins and heavy metals from the body.

It is also known for its quality for treating deadly viral and chronic bacterial infections. If combined with other natural herbs such as garlic clove, red clover blossom, cayenne and aloe vera, it can be extremely effective in cleaning your blood, skin, liver, and toxins present in the digestive system.

5. *Yarrow*: Yarrow is a powerful blood cleanser and helps in effective perspiration for a better waste removal. It is known for improving the health of glandular system and improves the function of liver. Yarrow can tone down mucous membrane of the intestines allowing better digestion.

Supplements for Detoxification: Vitamins and Minerals

Herbs are an important part of detoxification; however, the availability of herbs is a matter of concern and it is important to look out for other supplements. Vitamins and minerals play a crucial part in the overall health of the body and detoxification is one of the crucial functions they perform. The lymphatic system and liver require regular detoxification and here are some supplements that will help.

Supplements for liver detoxification

Most of the water-soluble toxins are excreted with urine and do not require special attention. However, fat-soluble toxins should be detoxified properly. Most of the detoxification processes takes place in the liver so, it is important to use supplements for its aid.

Some of the crucial supplements for liver detoxification include Vitamin A, Vitamin B1 & B6, Vitamin C, Vitamin E, Vitamin K, copper and biotin. These supplements work together with natural herbs for effective liver detoxification.

Lymph Detoxification

Lymph is responsible for washing blood and cells to get rid of any toxins. It is important to detoxify the lymphatic systems regularly with supplements such as Vitamin A, Vitamin B6, and vitamin C.

Role of antioxidants in detoxification

Regular exposure to toxins produce free radicals that are extremely dangerous for health. Free radicals can attack healthy body cells, weaken immune system, lead to premature aging of skin, and even cause cancer.

Antioxidants have a crucial role in terms of being the destroyer of free radicals and one can maintain sufficient antioxidants by taking Vitamin A, Vitamin C and Vitamin E, Copper, Selenium, Manganese and Zinc.

There is no doubt about the effectiveness of these vitamins and minerals in detoxification; however, it is important to include a weekly biking, running, or aerobic workout in your routine for overall detoxification.

Conclusion

An individual should create their own eating and working routine that supports cleansing and maintaining its natural detox ability. The trick is to balance the use of herbs, supplements, and physical workouts for a healthy body.

At the end of the day, it is better to figure out what works for you before trying out new methods in your quest to eliminate toxins. Do this a little at a time. Learning how to truly take care of yourself this way is already a great step towards a better well-being.

You will realize that the symptoms that plague you every day will go away almost instantly. The result is a better version of you.